HEALTH HELPERS

HOSPITAL WORKER

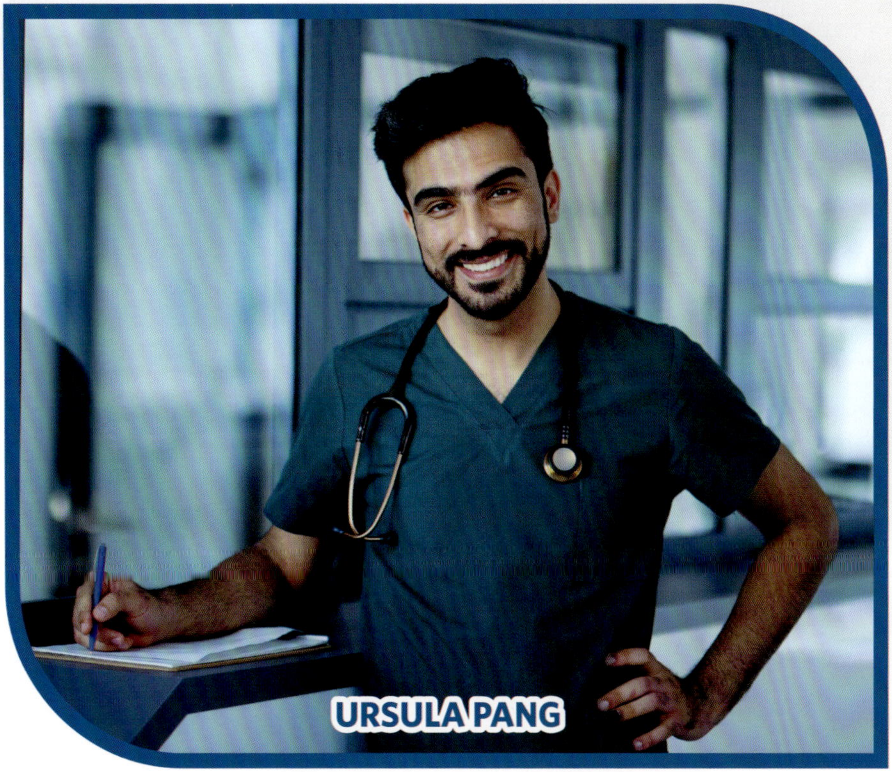

URSULA PANG

PowerKiDS press

Published in 2026 by The Rosen Publishing Group, Inc.
2544 Clinton Street, Buffalo, NY 14224

First Edition

Editor: Greg Roza
Book Design: Rachel Rising

Photo Credits: Cover, p. 1 Halfpoint/Shutterstock.com; pp. 4, 6, 8, 10, 12, 14, 16, 18, 20 TechSolution/Shutterstock.com; p. 5 New Africa/Shutterstock.com; p. 7 PeopleImages.com - Yuri A/Shutterstock.com; p. 9 Gorodenkoff/Shutterstock.com; p. 11 SofikoS/Shutterstock.com; p. 13 Peakstock/Shutterstock.com; p. 15 Media_Photos/Shutterstock.com; p. 17 DC Studio/Shutterstock.com; p. 19 Svitlana Hulko/Shutterstock.com; p. 21 Monkey Business Images/Shutterstock.com.

Names: Pang, Ursula.
Title: Hospital worker / Ursula Pang.
Description: Buffalo, New York : PowerKids Press, 2026. | Series: Health helpers | Includes glossary and index.
Identifiers: ISBN 9781499456523 (pbk.) | ISBN 9781499456530 (library bound) | ISBN 9781499456547 (ebook)
Subjects: LCSH: Hospitals–Employees–Juvenile literature. | Hospitals–Medical staff–Juvenile literature.
Classification: LCC RA972.P36 2026 | DDC 362.11068–dc23

Manufactured in China

CPSIA Compliance Information: Batch #QWPK26. For Further Information contact Rosen Publishing at 1-800-237-9932.

CONTENTS

Helpers at the Hospital 4
Doctors 6
Nurses 8
Working with Technology . . . 10
Therapists 12
Social Workers 14
Checking In 16
Feeling at Ease 18
Thanks, Hospital Helpers! 20
Glossary 22
For More Information 23
Index 24

Helpers at the Hospital

Have you ever been in a hospital? Maybe you were sick, or maybe you were visiting a sick family member. Having to stay in a hospital is no fun, but hospital workers of all kinds are there to help you get well. They are all health helpers!

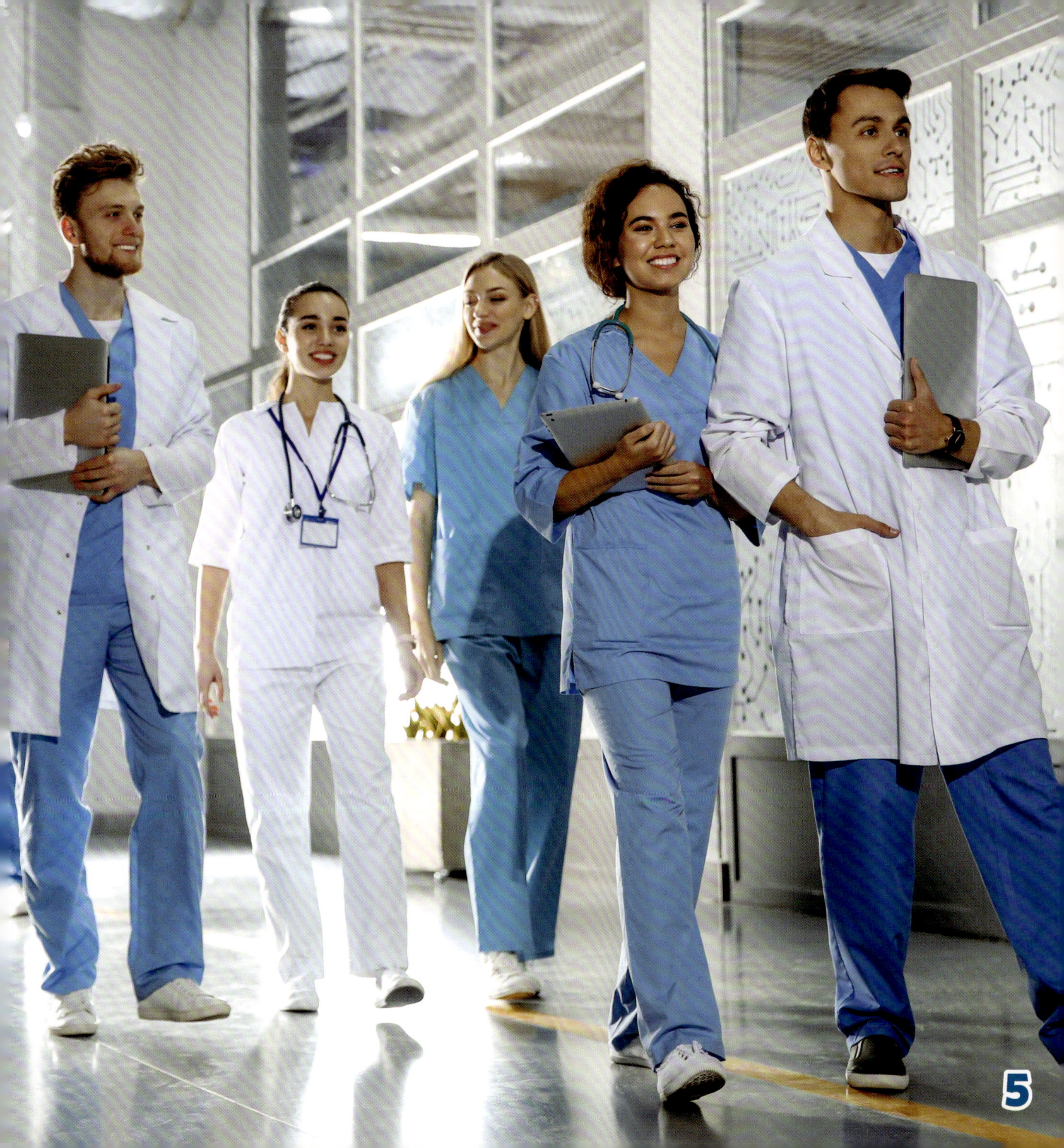

Doctors

The first hospital worker you may think of is a doctor. Many kinds of doctors work in hospitals. Some work with babies and children. Some doctors are **mental** health **experts**. Some hospital doctors are **surgeons**. One or more caring doctors will talk to you and treat your illness.

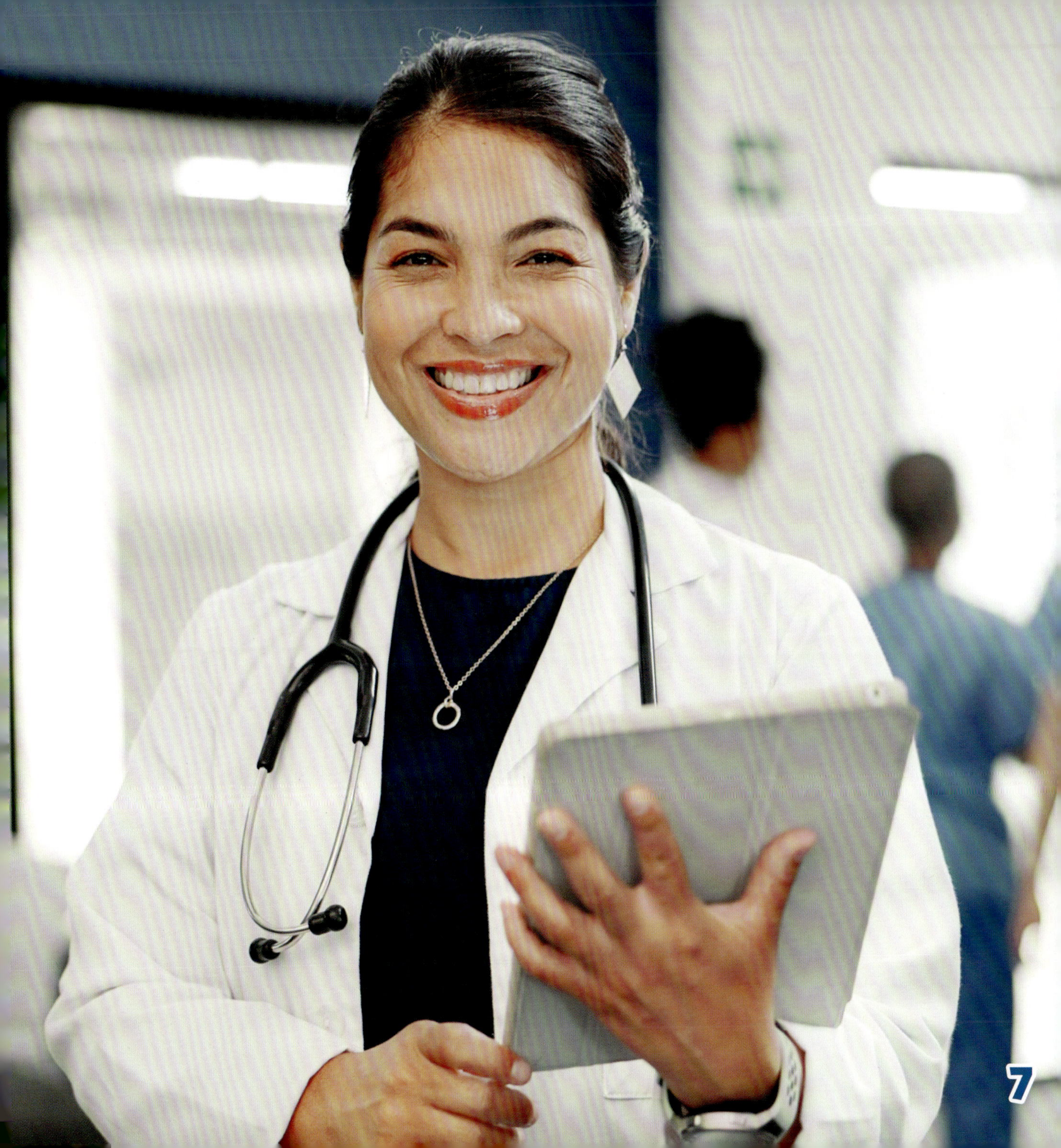

Nurses

Nurses are some of the busiest hospital workers. They keep close watch on **patients** and make sure they follow doctors' orders. They also make sure patients have what they need. Nurses give **medicine**. They change bandages. Some nurses are experts in taking blood from patients.

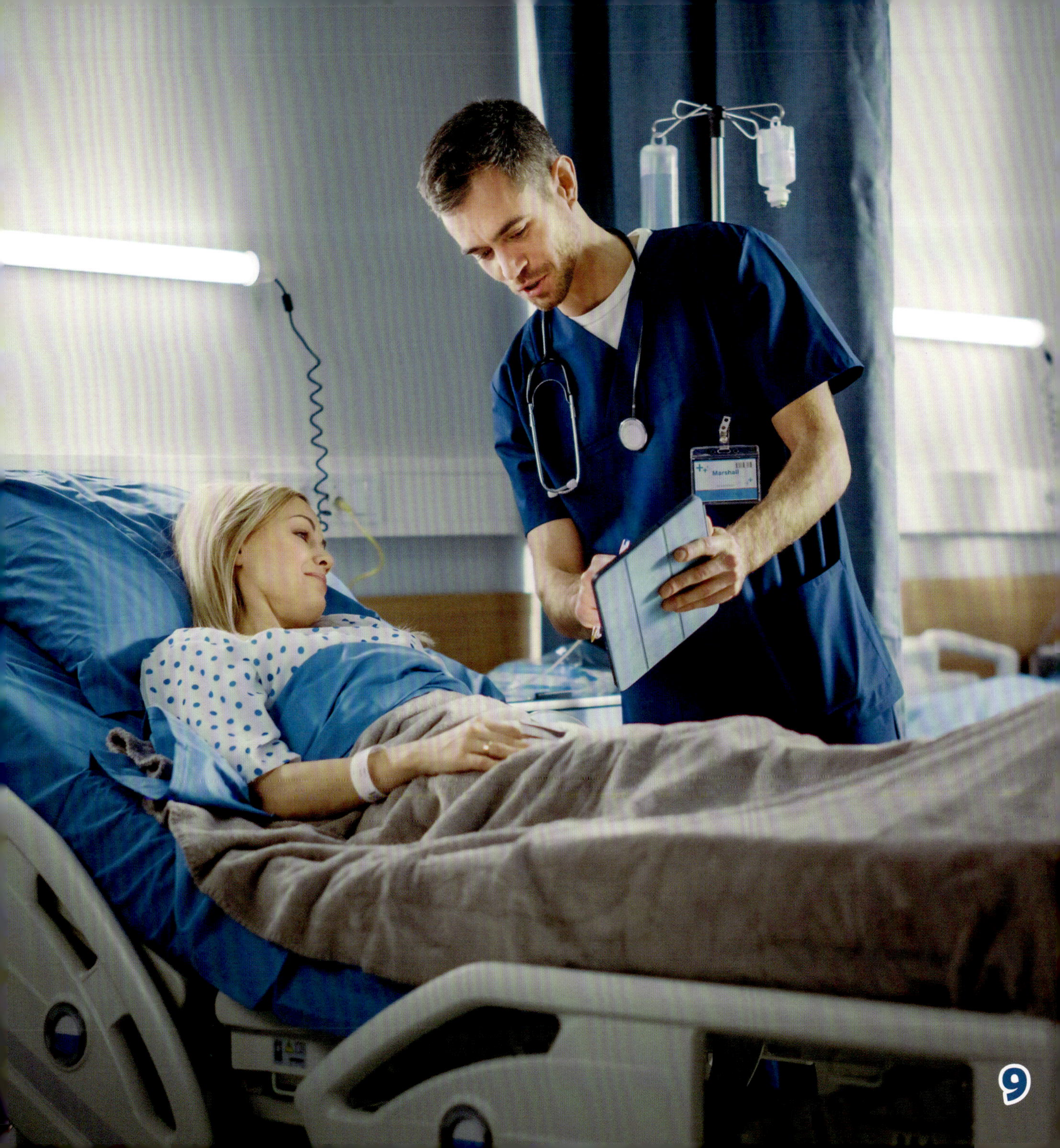
Marshall

Working with Technology

Hospitals need workers who know about **technology**, called technicians. You may not always see these workers. One technician you may see is the X-ray technician. That is a person trained to take X-rays. X-ray machines use waves of energy to see inside the body.

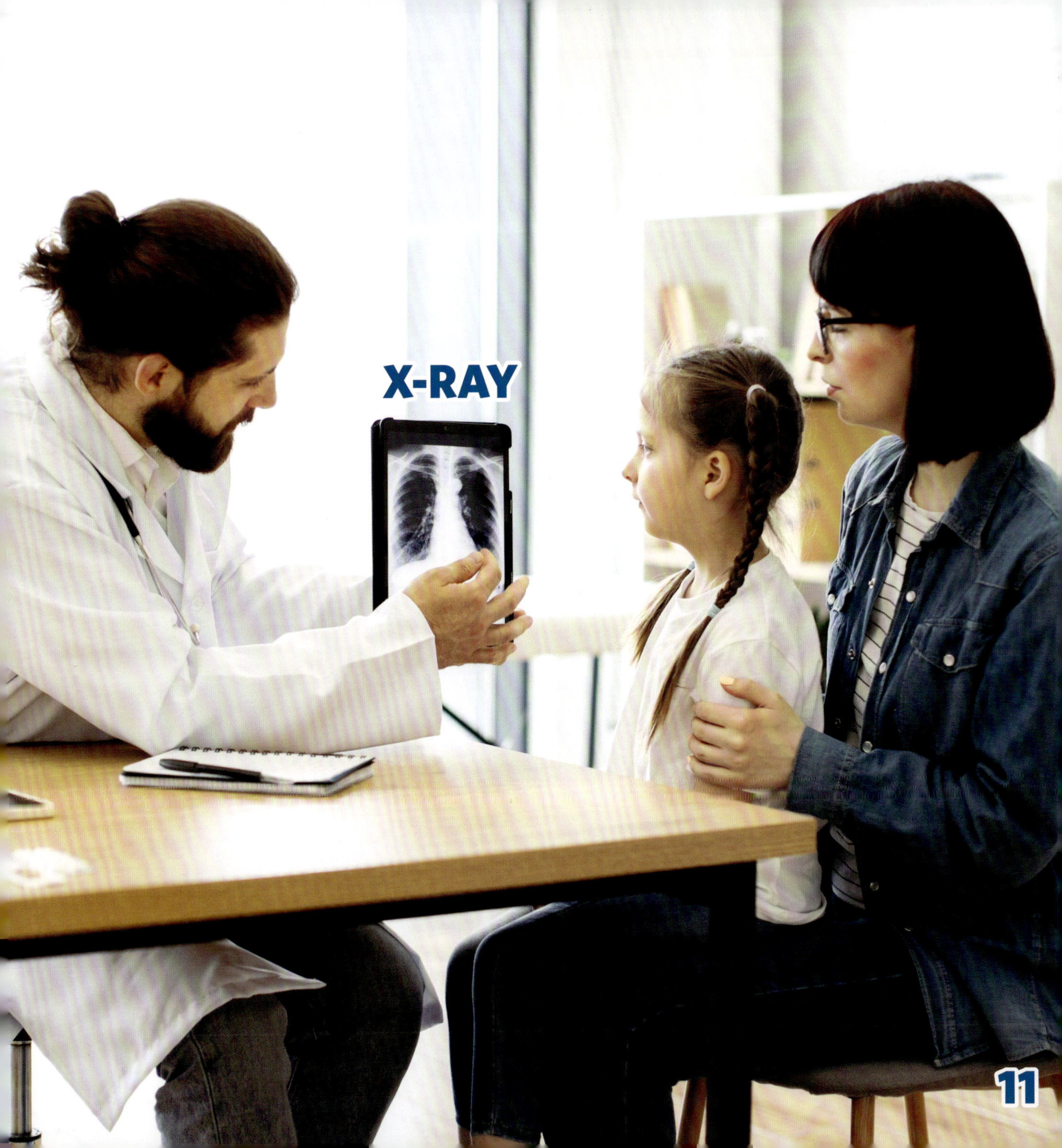
X-RAY

Therapists

Different kinds of therapists work in hospitals. Therapy is treatment used to make someone better. Physical therapists help patients recover from bodily injuries or illnesses. Some therapists help patients relearn life skills, such as cooking or getting dressed. Some hospitals even have therapy dogs!

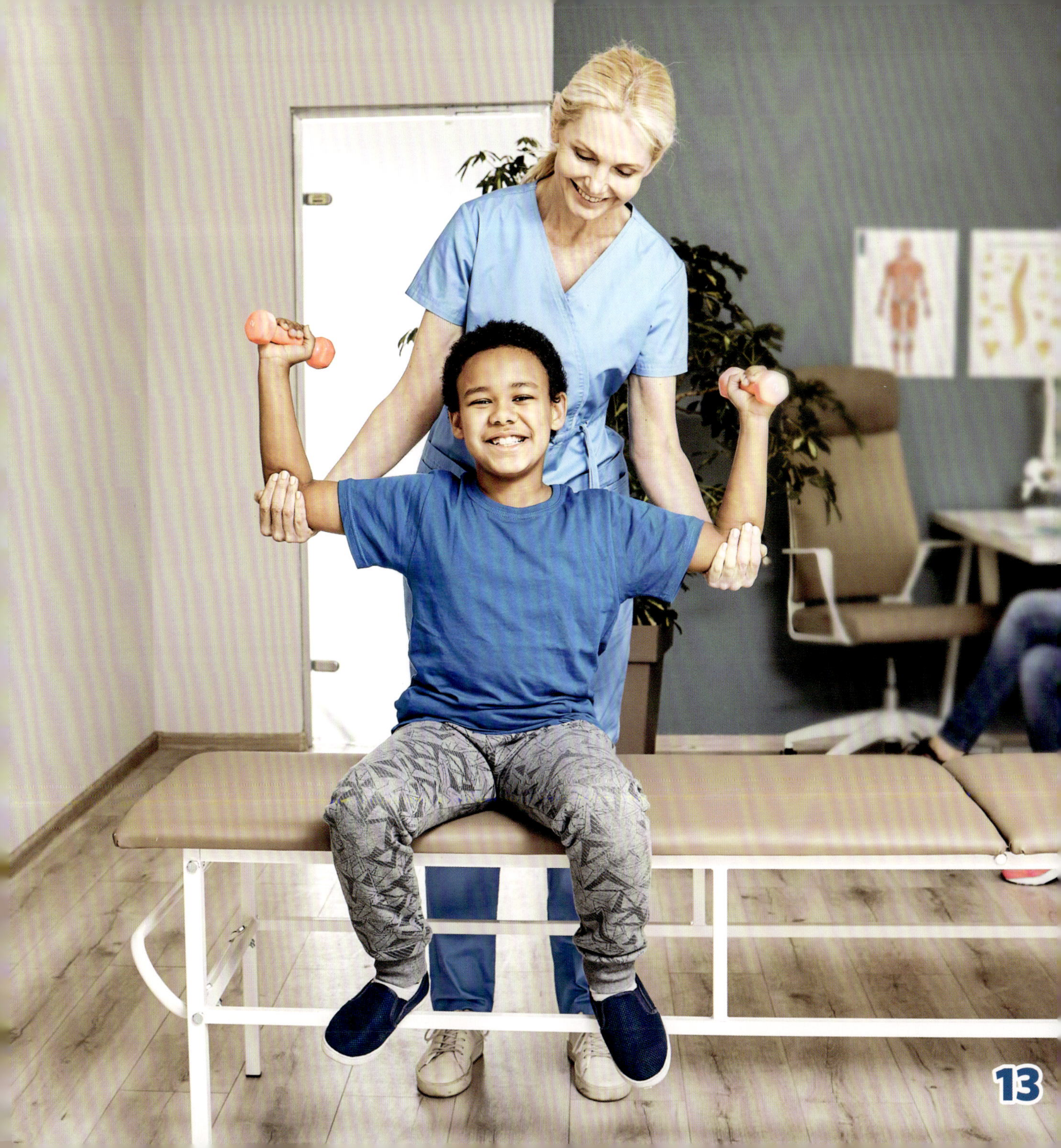

Social Workers

Hospital social workers give patients non-medical care. They help patients and their families cope with a stay in the hospital. They will help patients understand hospital practices. They give **emotional** support to worried families. They may also teach doctors and nurses how to deal with some patients' problems.

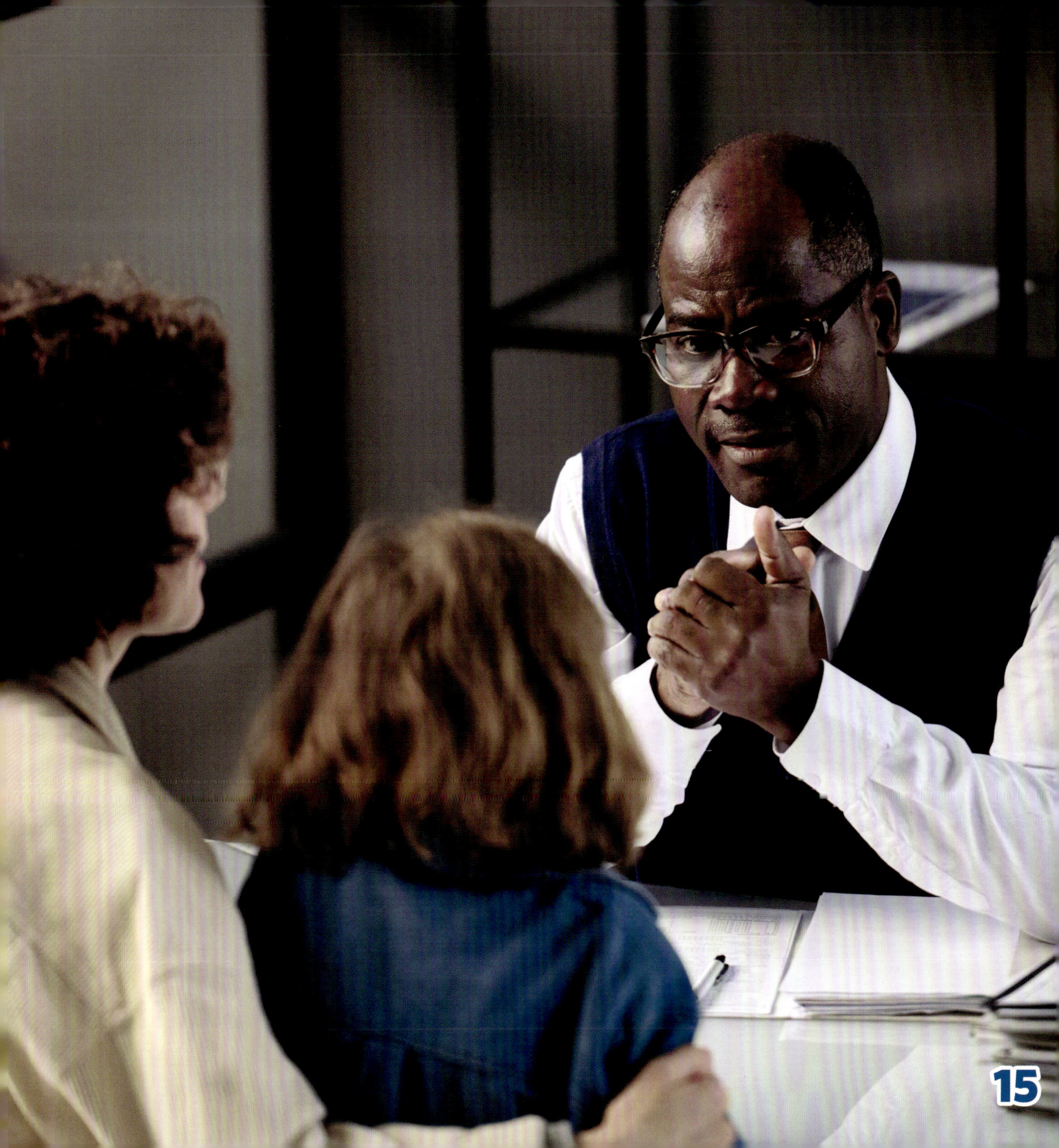

Checking In

Some hospital workers are there to help you check in and get where you need to go quickly. **Security** officers help you feel safe. Clerks take your information and get you signed in. Others keep track of medical records and make sure paperwork is correctly filled out.

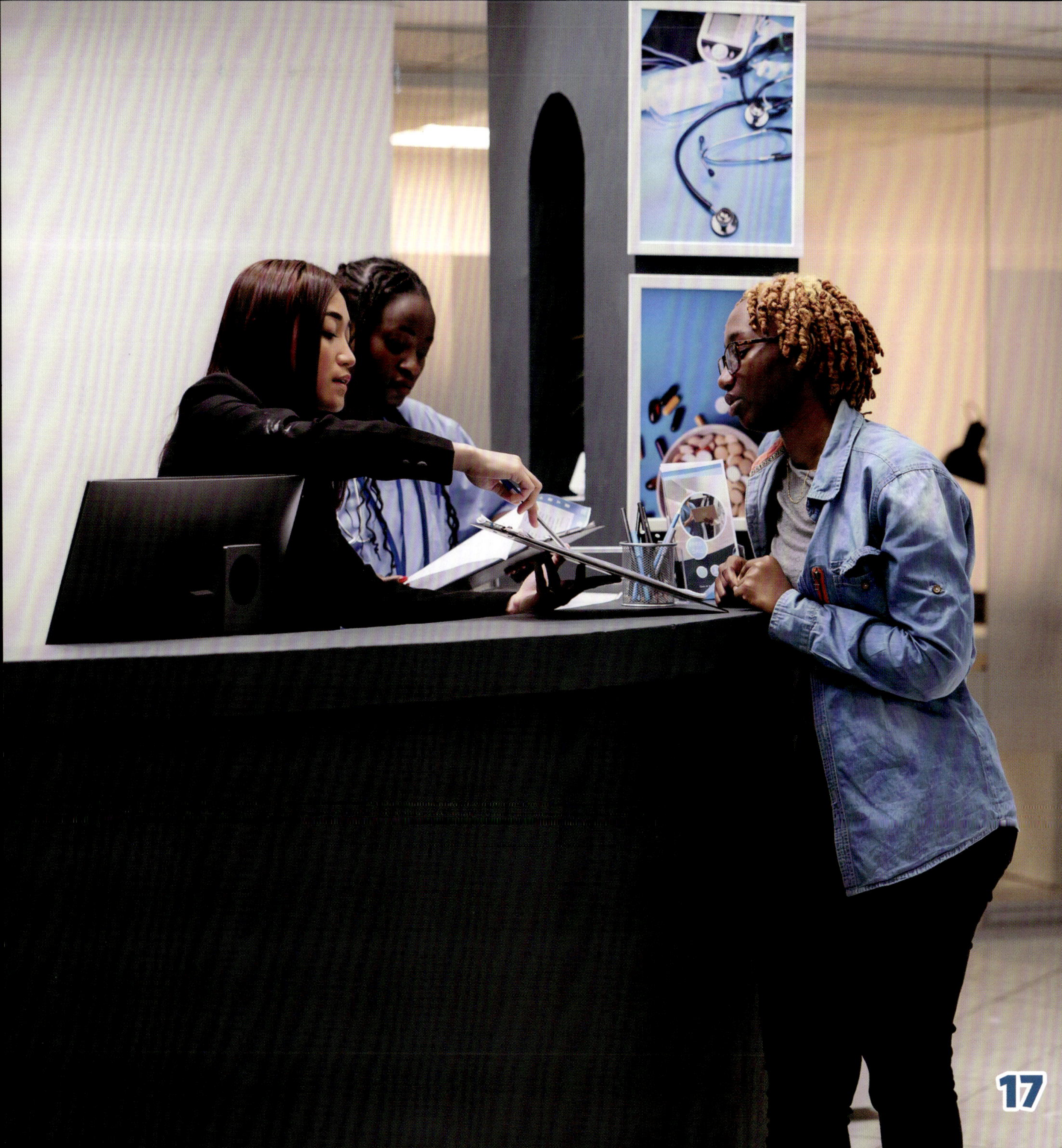

Feeling at Ease

Some hospital workers help make patients feel at ease. Orderlies are non-medical workers who help nurses do their job. They may help move patients from one bed to another. Many **janitors** help keep hospitals clean and germ free. Food service workers prepare meals for patients and hospital workers.

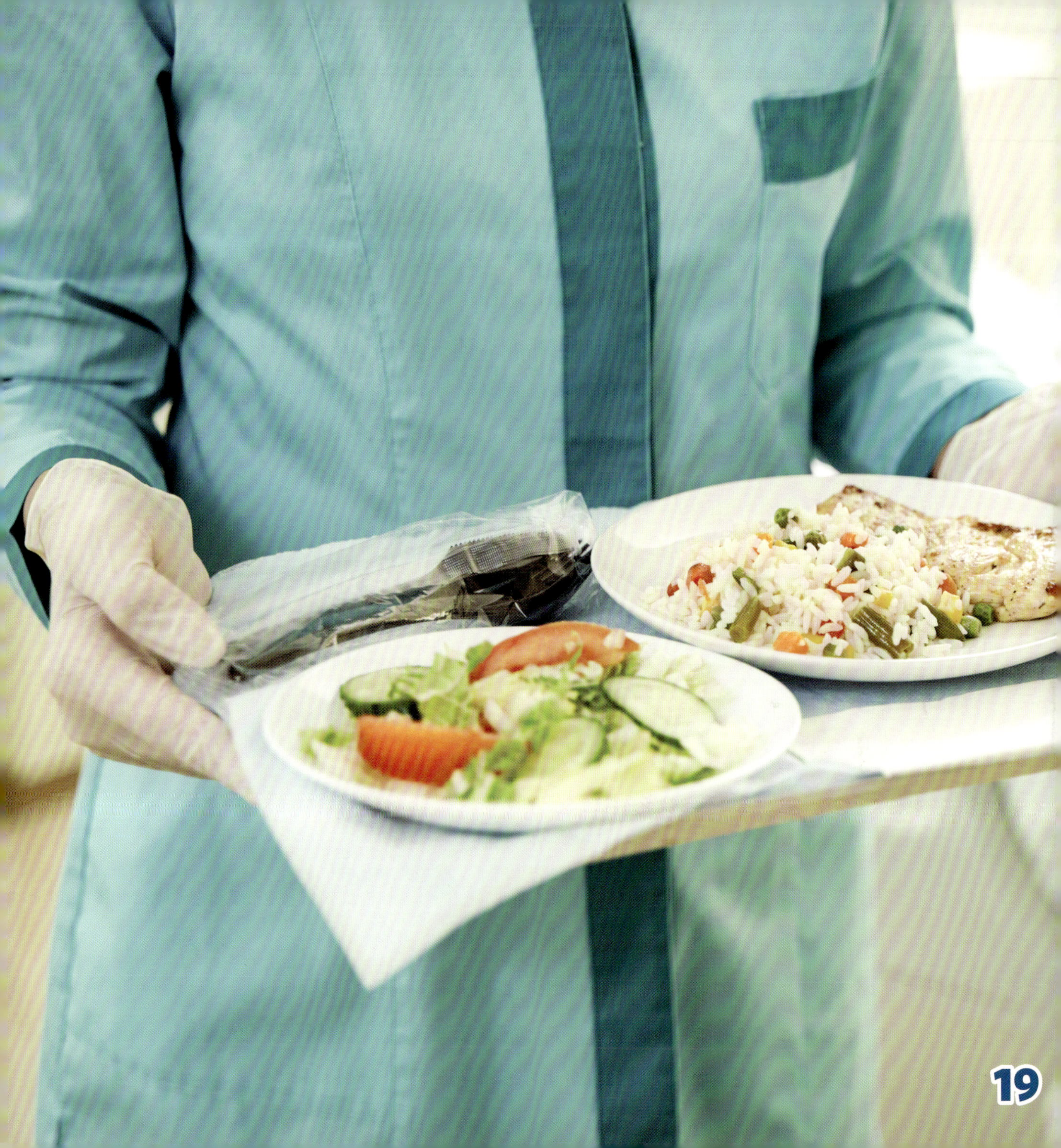

Thanks, Hospital Helpers!

Hospitals are filled with health helpers of many kinds. Some are trained to care for your health. Some are trained make your hospital stay simpler and easier. Some are trained to help you recover after an illness. Hospital workers make sure you and your family are healthy and happy!

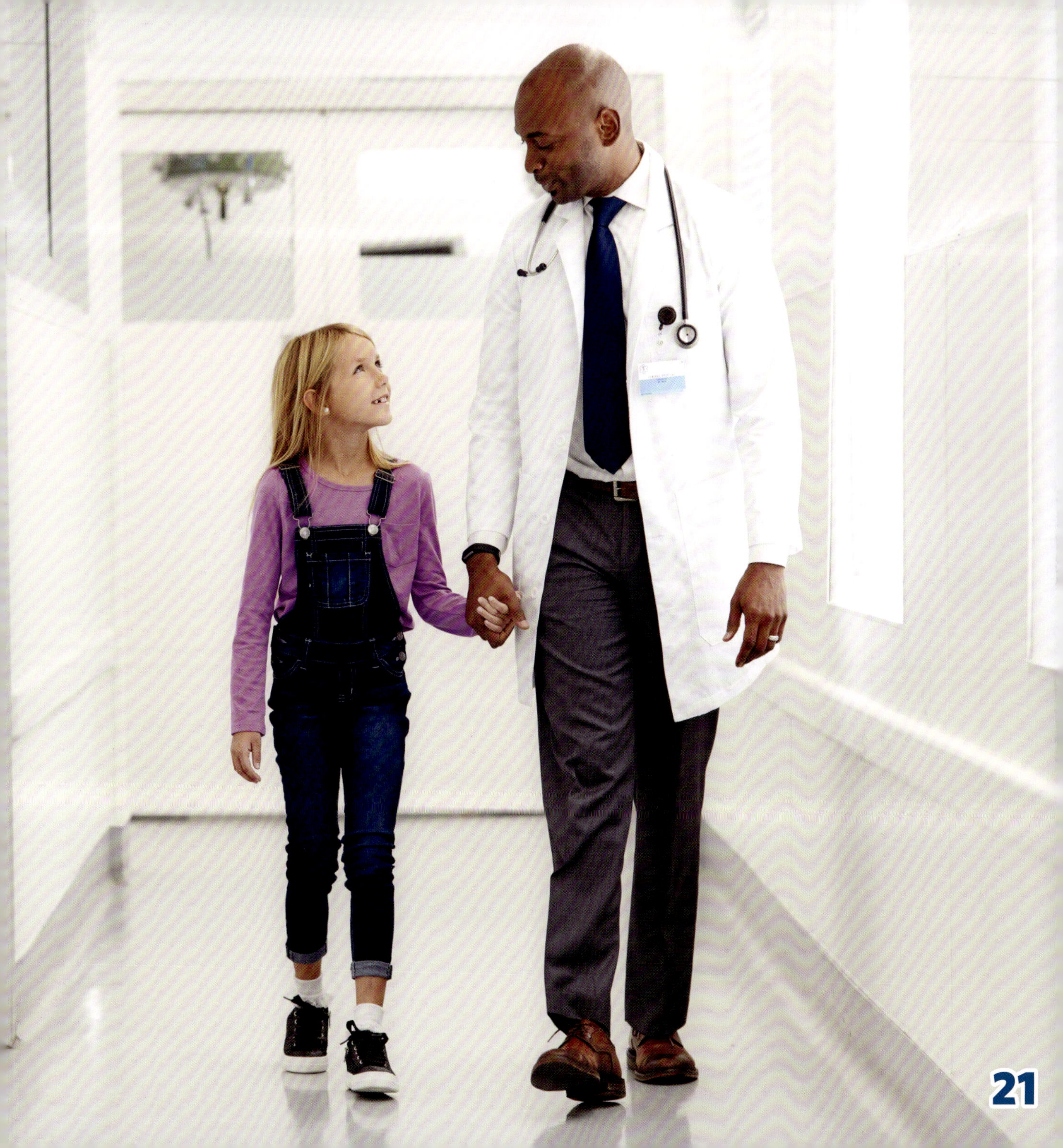

GLOSSARY

emotional: Having to do with feelings.

expert: Someone who knows a great deal about something.

janitor: Someone paid to clean a building.

medicine: A drug that a doctor gives you to help fight illness.

mental: Having to do with the mind.

patient: A person under medical care.

security: Having to do with safety.

surgeon: A doctor who treats people by cutting into the body.

technology: A method that uses science to solve problems and the tools used to solve those problems.

FOR MORE INFORMATION

BOOKS

Bolte, Mari. *Important Jobs in Hospitals*. Mankato, MN: Pebble Books, 2024.

Kukla, Lauren. *I'm a Doctor*. Rochester, MN: Mayo Clinic Press, 2024.

WEBSITES

Going to the Emergency Room
kidshealth.org/en/parents/emergency-room.html?ref=search
This webpage explains the A to Zs about the emergency room, from calling 911 to what happens after one leaves the ER.

Going to the Hospital
kidshealth.org/en/kids/hospital.html?ref=search
Kids Health walks readers though a stay at the hospital, including admissions, tests, doctors, and more.

Publisher's note to educators and parents: Our editors have carefully reviewed these websites to ensure that they are suitable for students. Many websites change frequently, however, and we cannot guarantee that a site's future contents will continue to meet our high standards of quality and educational value. Be advised that students should be closely supervised whenever they access the internet.

INDEX

C
clerks, 16

D
doctors, 6, 8, 14

F
food service workers, 18

J
janitors, 18

N
nurses, 8, 14, 18

O
orderlies, 18

P
patients, 8, 12, 14, 18

S
security, 16
social workers, 14

T
technicians, 10
therapists, 12